ACID REFLUX

Proven Methods to Cure Acid Reflux, Heartburn, and GERD

Anthony Wilkenson

Table of Contents

Important Insight

This book will give you a clear understanding of what acid reflux is – a health condition experienced by almost half of the American population. It explains how and why acid reflux occurs as well as discusses in detail why the common health remedies prescribed by health professionals do not eradicate the condition and worsen it instead. Much more than that, the book contains proven non-drug and non-surgical alternatives to effectively cure acid reflux, heartburn, and GERD.

Acid Reflux is a health condition where acidic stomach fluid leaks back up the food pipe (the esophagus) causing heartburn – a burning pain felt internally around the lower chest area. It is quite common for people to experience occasional heartburn since acid reflux usually results from eating or drinking certain types of food or drink for some people. However, the frequent occurrence of heartburn may indicate a more severe form of acid reflux condition called GERD (Gastro- Esophageal Reflux Disease). Although the condition may not be life threatening, it may lead to more serious health conditions in the future such as cancer if left unattended or uncared for. The book will help you eradicate the condition for good and prevent it from recurring without resorting to medication or surgery. I hope you find the information and recommendations truly valuable.

1: What Is Acid Reflux and Why do People Have It?

Acid reflux, also called GERD or Gastro-Esophageal Reflux Disease, is a condition where the acidic substance from the stomach flows back up into the esophagus or the food pipe. The back flow of stomach acid occurs if the lower esophageal sphincter fails to close properly.

The lower esophageal sphincter is a circular muscle located at the top of the stomach and acts as some sort of a gate valve that prevents stomach liquid from flowing back up into the esophagus. Normally, the lower esophageal sphincter contracts as soon as food is passed through it. However, there are times when it doesn't close tightly enough especially when it opens more frequently like when you go binge eating.

The sphincter needs to close or to constrict and must remain constricted all the time because once food gets into the stomach, the stomach walls start producing acid through the parietal cells to digest the food. This is part of the digestive process. The walls of the stomach are well adapted to the high level of acidity and are therefore adequately shielded from being harmed by the acid. Specifically, the mucous cells in the stomach walls produce enough mucous to coat the stomach walls entirely thus protecting them from the highly acidic, low ph environment of the stomach.

If the lower esophageal sphincter fails to close properly, a small amount of stomach acid flows back up into the esophagus irritating and inflaming its walls and produces that burning sensation. The walls of the esophagus are not like the stomach walls – they are not coated heavily with mucus. Over time, the constant and repeated flowing back of the acidic substance from the stomach up to the esophagus will ultimately damage the wall linings of the esophagus.

Every time these acidic substances from the stomach leaks and touches the linings of the esophagus it produces a burning sensation and other symptoms - which is actually our immune system's defensive reaction to the presence of acidic substance in the esophagus. In other words, these defensive reactions of the immune system which we now come to recognize as symptoms of acid reflux are our immune system's way of telling us there is an imbalance inside our body which needs to be corrected.

No one can really be quite certain what exactly causes the lower esophageal sphincter muscle to malfunction but there are a number of contributory risk factors which have been identified. The common symptoms or warning signs of acid reflux include heartburn, a discomfort or burning pain which moves from the stomach to the chest, abdomen, or throat; and regurgitation or bitter-tasting or sour acid which backs up in the mouth or throat.

The person may also experience bloating and gas after meals; black or bloody stools, or bloody vomiting; dysphagia or the narrowing of the esophagus which produces a food-stuck-in-the-throat sensation; feeling of extended fullness; burping, belching, gas, flatulence, rippling, gurgling sensations, frequent hiccups, nausea, weight loss for no apparent reason; chronic sore throat, hoarseness, persistent dry cough, or wheezing; erosion of tooth enamel, diarrhea, and constipation.

Let me emphasize once again - these symptoms are urgent warning signs that must not be ignored. They are telling us something's wrong inside our bodies – specifically there is a digestive dysfunction that is causing an imbalance inside the body that needs to be corrected. This point needs emphasis because as you will later on find out - the standard approach taken by most health care specialists in managing acid reflux is to suppress the symptoms through medication. However, symptomatic relief via medications in effect only worsens the patient's condition. At best, their approach merely provides temporary respite from the pain and sufferings due to the symptoms - but does not address much less eliminate the real cause or causes of acid reflux.

If you remember what we've said earlier - it is the lower esophageal sphincter muscle which acts as a one-way gate valve that opens automatically to allow food to enter the stomach and then closes promptly to prevent the acidic content of the stomach to flow back into the esophagus. It means acid reflux (*the flowing back of stomach acid up the esophagus*) can only happen if the lower esophageal sphincter muscle "relaxes" or becomes weak or loosens up - preventing it from constricting fully. It means the lower esophageal sphincter muscle is unable to function properly – staying open when it has to be closed or constricted.

In this context, we can safely say that the onslaught of acid reflux symptoms may vary in severity according to 3 things:

- The muscular tone of the lower esophageal sphincter muscle - a weaker LES muscle will leave a bigger opening allowing more stomach acid to flow back.

- The level of acidity and pH of the liquid flowing back into the esophagus.

- The ability of the esophagus muscles to naturally cleanse the impurities that may have accumulated at the bottom of the esophagus – the impurities can lead to infection of the LES muscle which may weaken it.

According to a recent study, about 60% of the population experiences acid reflux symptoms (*particularly heart burn or pyrosis – another name for heart burn*) at least once within a year. About 20% to 30% of the population experiences the symptoms on a weekly basis. Based on another survey, people who experience GERD symptoms on a weekly basis have been affected by these symptoms for five years. The number of people who were diagnosed with primary and secondary Gastro-Esophageal Reflux Disease has also dramatically risen by a whopping 216% from 995,402 in 1998 to 3,141,965 in 2005.

According to the American College of Gastroenterology, there are at least 60 million Americans who suffer from heartburn monthly. About 15 million Americans experience heartburn daily. In the December 2011 issue of the Gut journal, a study was published which said that there are 50% more acid reflux sufferers than there were some 10 years ago.

The question now is who are at risk? Who are the people most likely to suffer from GERD or Gastro-Esophageal Reflux Disease? More important – what puts people at risk of developing acid reflux?

2: Who is at Risk of Having Acid Reflux?

About 60% of the population experience acid reflux symptoms at least once a year, a number of them are simply normal, natural reactions to certain food or drink these people may have recently drank or consumed. We are least interested with the intermittent, infrequent occurrence of acid reflux symptoms among these people as it does not necessarily indicate the presence of GERD or gastro-esophageal reflux disease. What we are more interested in is how many of these acid reflux sufferers repeatedly experience the symptoms with greater frequency – the experience becoming more regular and more pronounced as the days passes by.

The recurrence of the acid reflux symptoms indicates that the gastro-esophageal reflux disease has set in and that the walls of the esophagus are starting to feel the damage by the onslaught of acid reflux. Left unchecked, the acid reflux disease can lead to more serious health conditions which are even more difficult to manage. To effectively manage and possibly totally eradicate acid reflux we must be able to recognize the onslaught of the disease early on. However, this is easier said than done because even doctors have difficulty determining why their patients have the gastro-esophageal reflux disease. With a myriad of aggravating factors each of which can produce severe and painful acid reflux symptoms, one would really be hard put to pin down the real reason why a person has the acid reflux disease.

We know for a fact that acid reflux occurs because the lower esophageal sphincter muscle (LES) has weakened substantially to a point that it is unable to close properly after food has passed through it. However, we also know for a fact that there is not just one but several aggravating factors that can weaken the LES muscle and predispose people to the onslaught of the acid reflux disease.

First and foremost of these aggravating factors is a stomach abnormality called hiatal hernia. Hiatal hernia is an abnormal genetic condition where the diaphragm – *the muscle wall that separates the stomach from the chest* – is too weak to hold the LES muscle and the upper part of the stomach in place thus allowing the LES muscle and the upper part of the stomach to move up above the diaphragm (see the illustration on the right). This makes it easier for stomach acid to flow back up into the esophagus as a result. What complicates matters more is the fact that sometimes people with this type of stomach abnormality do not show signs of acid reflux until it is too late.

A person diagnosed with hiatal hernia may experience vomiting, nausea, or severe pain in the abdomen or chest. He may also be unable to move his bowels or pass gas. In this case what he has is strangulated hernia which becomes an obstruction. He must call a doctor as soon as possible because it is a medical emergency.

Immediate surgery through laparoscopy is usually recommended for para-esophageal hernia because the stomach can be strangulated. Laparoscopic surgery has lesser risk of scarring, pain, and infection. Furthermore, the patient can also quickly recover from it. He can also be up and about a day after the procedure. He may go back to his normal routine within a week. He is considered completely recovered within 3 weeks.

Pregnancy in women is also another aggravating factor that leads to acid reflux. The increased hormone levels during pregnancy plus the growing fetus often forces acidic stomach liquid to flow back up into the esophagus producing acid reflux symptoms in the process. Many women in fact experience acid reflux symptoms for the first time during their pregnancy. Good news is the symptoms go away after they delivered their babies.

Acid reflux symptoms like abdominal pain, bloating, belching, intestinal gas, indigestion or heartburn may also be an indication of an overgrowth of Candida Albicans in the colon. Candida is a type of fungus (or yeast) small amounts of which live and are always present in our digestive system – particularly the mouth and intestines. Candida helps with digestion and nutrient absorption but their numbers are held in check by the good bacteria. However, there are certain conditions when Candida is overproduced – like when antibiotics you have taken kill some of the good bacteria disrupting the balance allowing Candida to grow unabated.

Other factors that promote Candida overgrowth include high alcohol intake, diets high in refined carbohydrates and sugar (they serve as food for the yeast), oral contraceptives or any number of other factors including a high-stress lifestyle. An overgrowth of Candida results in the breakdown of the intestinal walls allowing the Candida to penetrate the bloodstream where it starts releasing toxic byproducts causing leaky gut.

It is a widely accepted fact that acid reflux originates in the colon and results from years and years of a fungal yeast infection that builds up in the colon.

When Candida Albicans turn from yeast to fungi, they produce more than 79 distinct toxins. These toxins are responsible for many of the symptoms that Candida sufferers have including heartburn. Candida overgrowth results in their fermentation which in turn results in refluxing the contents of the stomach upwards straight through the small intestines, into the stomach and finally into the esophagus where they cause infection, inflammation, burning sensation and damage to the esophagus.

There are also certain lifestyle factors that predispose people to the risk of acid reflux disease. Smoking is one of these lifestyle factors that can lead to GERD. Nicotine and a number of other harmful elements from cigarette smoking damage the mucus membranes of the throat and impair muscle reflexes. Smoking also induces increased secretion of acid which further impairs the proper functioning of the lower esophageal sphincter. Salivation is also reduced which in effect limits the natural process of neutralizing acid by the saliva. And, if smoking is combined with heavy alcohol drinking, the immune system is weakened further increasing the risk of developing cancer of the esophagus.

Eating and/or drinking certain food and beverages that are known to induce acid reflux symptoms is another lifestyle factor that predisposes people to the acid reflux disease. Some of these acid reflux foods are carbonated drinks, alcohol, chocolate, eating large meals or lying down right after a meal can trigger heartburn or other symptoms of acid reflux disease, such as a dry cough or trouble swallowing. These are some of the common acid reflux foods that trigger symptoms:

Carbonated beverages, Coffee or tea (regular or decaffeinated), Fatty or fried foods, spicy foods, such as those containing chili or curry, Foods containing tomato, such as spaghetti sauce, salsa, or pizza, citrus fruits, such as oranges or lemons, mint, garlic and onions.

Lack of nutrition is also another mitigating factor. We depend more on processed foods and less and less on natural foods which have high nutritional value. As a consequence, our immune system weakens making it easier for Candida to grow unhampered and cause digestive problems as well as aggravate acid reflux condition.

Over-acidity in the digestive system is another mitigating factor. Over-acidity thickens the blood and make them sludgy thus producing an environment which is ideal for Candida overgrowth. Over-acidity results from having a diet high in acidic foods resulting in a more acidic stomach.

Sluggish digestion is also a major factor. A sluggish digestive system means undigested food and rotten food particles gets stored in the digestive tract much longer than necessary allowing further Candida overgrowth which in turn results in acid reflux.

Stress due to pressure in your daily routine, emotional issues, inadequate sleep, or anxiety have been known to weaken the immune system and trigger digestive problems. Stress results in elevated blood sugar levels providing Candida cells with food to grow. Ultimately, Candida becomes the more dominant bacteria resulting in the aggravation of acid reflux.

Obesity is also a mitigating factor. With more fat cells putting pressure on your abdomen and clogging up your middle, the harder it is for the digestive system to function properly. Intense pressure on the abdomen results in the acidic stomach content being refluxed into the esophagus where it can cause more damage.

A person may also experience symptoms of the acid reflux disease if he lies down immediately after eating or eats large portions of meals, is obese or overweight, bends over at the waist or lie on his back after eating a heavy meal, or snacks before he sleeps. Taking blood pressure medicines, some muscle relaxants, ibuprofen, or aspirin may also induce acid reflux symptoms particularly heartburn.

Dietary Choices, over-acidity and sluggish digestion, stress, Inadequate Sleep, obesity, over acidity, Candida over growth – altogether they all contribute in creating an internal imbalance and promotes a perfect environment for the formation and aggravation of acid reflux.

3: How Do You Know for Sure you have Acid Reflux?

If the symptoms occur at least twice a week, it is time for the person to visit a doctor for a thorough diagnosis. It is not advisable to take self-prescribed medicines to alleviate the suffering from the symptoms because as you will learn in the later chapters, this will only worsen the condition. On the other hand, seeing a doctor does not guarantee that you will know for sure what is ailing you. In the first place, as we said earlier, even doctors have difficulty determining for sure which one among the many mitigating factors is causing you to experience the pain and discomfort of the acid reflux disease.

Unless a thorough diagnosis is made, a doctor is reduced to determining the cause on a trial and error basis – prescribing medicines to alleviate your suffering for the symptoms you happen to complain about. Only when the symptoms are serious enough will the doctor order a thorough diagnosis which may include the following tests.

- An esophagram or Barium Swallow Radiograph to check for the narrowing of the esophagus or ulcers. The patient will be required to swallow a solution so that the internal structures will be visible on the X-ray machine.

- The Esophageal Manometry, on the other hand, will check if the lower esophageal sphincter and esophagus are functioning normally.

- The doctor may also check the pH level of the esophagus by inserting a device and leaving it there for at most 2 days in order to measure the presence of acid in the esophagus. This is the most common and standard diagnostic test for acid reflux. It makes use of a thin wire with an acid sensor which is inserted through the nose all the way down into the lower area of the esophagus. The pH probe is attached to a monitoring device worn outside the body. You are then monitored for 24-hour periods to determine if the acidity levels of your esophagus alters during each meal, during activities and while you sleep

- An endoscopy may also be ordered if the doctor suspects more serious problems in the stomach or esophagus. It will require a lighted, flexible, and long tube to be inserted down the throat. The doctor may sedate the person and spray the throat with anesthesia to make him more comfortable.

- Lastly, a doctor may perform a biopsy during endoscopy to take tissue samples to test for abnormalities or infection.

The Barium Swallow Radiograph is used to rule out any problems with the esophagus structure. It is painless as the person is made to swallow a barium solution. This method can only diagnose about 1/3 of all the GERD cases because not all GERD sufferers have changes in their esophagus which can be clearly identified by X-rays. An EGD or Endoscopy requires a small tube with a camera to be inserted through the mouth so that the doctor can see the lining of the stomach and esophagus. A sedative is administered by the gastroenterologist before the tube is inserted. An analgesic may be sprayed on the throat so that the person becomes more comfortable during the process.

The test may take about 20 minutes. It won't block the air passages so he won't have any difficulty breathing. It also isn't painful. The process may detect GERD complications like Barrett's esophagus and esophagitis. However, only about 50% of individuals suffering from GERD may be diagnosed because not all have experienced changes in their esophagus lining. The biopsy is performed, depending on the results of the endoscopy. The gastroenterologist uses a surgical instrument to get a small portion of the esophagus lining, which is then sent for analysis to the pathology laboratory. The tissue is most often checked for esophageal cancer.

4: Conventional Treatment of the Acid Reflux Disease

Conventional medicine has a wide array of medications to deal with acid reflux – a great number of them are over-the-counter products. The problem is none of them have been able to effectively eliminate the acid reflux disease much less totally eradicate the symptoms associated with the disease in the long run. This is mainly because most of these medications, particularly the over-the-counter medicines, are limited to alleviating specific symptoms associated the acid reflux disease. They do not address the root cause of the acid reflux disease.

There are in fact some conventional anti-acidic treatments that can effectively alleviate the symptoms. However, there are two caveats to that treatment everyone must put in mind:

- They merely provide temporary symptomatic relief. Reflux is a complex condition and treatment must be holistic. To effectively eliminate it the environment that keeps it alive must be neutralized. For example, reducing the inflammation in the esophagus is just like cutting the plant but leaving the roots in the soil. It will definitely recur again.

- All acid reflux medications also carry a myriad of side effects, some of which are serious.

People often resort to using over-the-counter drugs when there is a sudden and aggravated onset of the acid reflux disease that requires immediate or instant relief. Sadly however, there is a dark side to the OTCs - they may offer temporary relief but they actually aggravate the condition in the long run as they irritate your stomach or esophagus lining. Known side effects of some of these prescription drugs are even life threatening such as severe ulcers and stomach bleeding. As a rule you should avoid OTC medication for acid reflux.

For the sake of educating you about available conventional treatments and over-the-counter acid reflux medications, here is a list of these products and their effect on acid reflux:

Antacids

Antacids are drugs aimed at neutralizing stomach acid by emptying the acid from the stomach. In this way the reflux liquid will contain no acid. Although antacids work very fast, their effect is quickly reduced as acid re-accumulates in the stomach. Antacids are most effective if taken either just before eating or an hour after a meal. This way, it lingers longer in the stomach potentially increasing its effect.

Neutralizing acid stomach is done using three basic salts –magnesium, calcium, and aluminum – mixed with hydroxide or bicarbonate ions.

The problem with calcium-based antacids is that they also stimulate the release of a hormone called gastrin that is mainly responsible for stimulating the production of stomach acid, which is counterproductive. Antacids also have some side effects including nausea, diarrhea, and constipation.

Pepto Bismol

Pepto Bismol is a famous antacid OTC product that may temporarily soothe acid reflux and IBS (irritable bowel syndrome) symptoms, help digestion and ease nausea. Pepto Bismol contains aspirin and bismuth subsalicylate - an active ingredient that impedes the growth of bacteria, particularly H. pylori. Pepto Bismol can cause side effects such as ringing in the ears.

Foaming Agents

A very popular medicine for heartburn, Gaviscon is an over-the-counter drug. Gaviscon contains alginic acid and is different than most antacid drugs. Alginate drugs vary in composition but they have antacid in their formula. The acid works by developing a barrier against the acid in the stomach - done by creating a foamy gel on top of the gastric pool. It refluxes past the sphincter harmlessly.

The most active ingredient in alginate drugs is also naturally found in brown algae. Foaming agents are drugs that help cover your stomach contents with foam to prevent acid reflux. They contain a combination of aluminum hydroxide gel, magnesium trisilicate and alginate. Foaming agents are best taken after meals and in combination with other drugs to maximize their effectiveness. If your esophagus is damaged, foaming agents are useless.

H2 Blockers

H2 blockers (histamine antagonists) suppress acid production by attaching themselves to the receptor cells in the stomach. H2 blockers blocks type 2 histamines preventing them from stimulating the production of acid. If you suffer from inflammation in the esophagus, H2 blockers are useless, but they can be effective at temporarily alleviating the symptoms of GERD. The only difference between over-the-counter H2 blockers and those that are prescribed by doctors is the strength of the drug or the dosage.

Proton Pump Inhibitors (PPIs)

Proton-pump inhibitors such as Zantac are often prescribed to GERD sufferers to provide immediate relief for heartburn. PPIs reduce the effect of the acid reflux by blocking acid production in the stomach. Zantac was the first proton-pump inhibitor prescribed to help GERD patients.

Other proton-pump inhibitors that may be prescribed by the gastroenterologist can include rabeprazole (Aciphex brand), omeprazole (Prilosec; may be bought without prescription), dexlansoprazole (Dexilant), esomeprazole (Nexium), lansoprazole (Prevacid), pantoprazole (Protonix), and omeprazole with sodium bicarbonate (Zegerid).

In general, these medicines are effective and safe. However, they may cause side effects and may not be appropriate for everyone. Proton pump inhibitors are more potent than H2 blockers, and their success rate at alleviating the symptoms of GERD are definitely higher. PPIs work by blocking the production of acid in your stomach while helping your esophagus heal from inflammation since they shield it against any contact with acidic reflux. PPIs are usually used when H2 blockers prove to be ineffective. They are best taken before meals.

Prokinetics

Prokinetics, also called pro-motility drugs, are aimed at helping your stomach expel content more rapidly, enhance the stomach muscle tone and strengthen the LES. Prokinetics are most effective when taken before meals and at bedtime. However, prokinetics can cause some side effects and are not helpful at treating complications of GERD or at relieving the symptoms of acid reflux.

If your heartburn does not improve with lifestyle changes, OTCs or drugs, you may need additional tests such as barium swallow radiograph, pH monitoring, endoscopy and biopsy, and you may be advised by your doctor to undergo the following procedures:

Surgery

Surgery should only be considered when no improvement has been made using OTCs or through the treatment of drugs. Surgery is crucial in cases where the regurgitation is severe and chronic. These are cases which cannot be treated by drugs and often results in lung infection. Some reflux sufferers opt for surgery instead of taking a large volume of drugs needed to control their symptoms. Doctors may often recommend surgery when Barrett's esophagus occurs to eliminate GERD and to prevent cancerous growth in the esophagus.

5: The Medical Paradigm and the Sad Truth about Conventional Medicines

The sad truth about conventional medicines is that they all have side effects – a dirty little secret they want to keep under wraps. Apparently they want to keep it that way. What we see today is a medical paradigm where the medical profession and the pharmaceutical industries do not seem to want to find a cure for the various diseases that afflict man.

Pharmaceutical companies make drugs that address only one set of symptoms and sell them with the knowledge that prolonged use of these drugs will cause a new set of medical problems. The drug companies then produce new medications to solve the new set of medical problems spawned by the use of the first drug. The medial profession on the other hand continues to prescribe these drugs with full knowledge that they may lead to more serious side effects.

As for you, you are kept in the dark. What happens is when you start taking a drug prescribed by your doctor for a particular symptom you currently have, you are totally clueless that sometime in the future you will develop a new medical condition resulting from its use. When the new medical condition occurs a few months later, you won't realize that it was actually caused by the first drug you took!

However, your doctor is fully aware of this and is likely going to give you another drug for the new medical condition. Definitely the new drug will alleviate the symptoms and may appear to work - but again a new series of medical problems will once again develop a few months later. This becomes a vicious cycle with no end in sight – albeit a profitable one for both the pharmaceutical companies and the health professionals.

The disturbing truth is that the medical establishment and the pharmaceutical companies seem to simply want to continue to sell drugs that merely alleviate the symptoms neglecting or toning down the search for the cures. That way we will always be needy for new medicines and end up spending more money while they (the pharmaceutical companies and the health professionals) make more profit as we find ourselves. It doesn't make sense to us but it does to them – after all, it is all about money.

Another disturbing truth is the tendency of Western medicine to classify many illnesses as genetic disorders. This erroneously leads us to believe that we are born with a certain disease and that there is nothing we can do to remedy the situation but merely seek relief for the symptoms.

The truth however is that even if we are born with certain genetic weaknesses, we have the capacity to control our own health and well-being. Our body has a built-in capacity to heal itself. It is a remarkable system for self-repair that works 24/7 - day in and day out. The best part is improving our ability for self-healing is within our control.

Unfortunately, not too many people are able to grasp the body's incredible power to heal itself from any illness. We have been dependent on traditional Western medicine far too long that we believe good health comes from outside the body. It surely will surprise you to know that if just left alone, 50 percent of all illnesses will eventually heal - all by themselves.

Every single moment of our existence, every single cell in our body are endlessly working to bring us back to a natural state of equilibrium or homeostasis. Each cell is constantly monitoring its own processes - endlessly working to maintain internal stability and balance as well as to continuously restore itself to the original DNA code it was born with. Our cells have the capacity to not only heal themselves but to reproduce new cells as well that will replace those that have been damaged or destroyed permanently. Even if a large cluster of cells is damaged or destroyed, the surrounding cells will immediately replicate creating new cells in the process to replace the cells that were destroyed. , thereby replacing almost immediately.

What we only need to do is understand the internal problem that caused the disease, listen to what our body needs, take full control over our health and making the necessary lifestyle changes adopt proper dietary regimens and undertake internal cleansing. This is the only way we can regain our health and take full control of our life without worrying about the cost much less the side effects of traditional Western medicines.

6: The Best Cure Is No Cure at All

That is right. Because our body strives every single day to automatically heal itself, there is no need for us to resort to taking medications for whatever it is that bothers us. The only thing we need to do to get our body to begin healing itself is to remove the barriers to healing which we have placed there ourselves. It will be a big mistake to think that taking medicines will fast track the body's self-healing processes because in reality they only serve as barriers that prevent the healing process from taking its natural course - particularly when side-effects of the drugs starts to pop up.

Besides, conventional medicines are meant to suppress and counteract the symptoms of the disease for which they were prescribed. Don't forget that the symptoms are vital signals produced by the immune system to tell the body that there is an internal imbalance that has to be corrected. These signals are part and parcel of the body's self healing process.

By suppressing, the symptoms, you are in effect denying the immune system to send out signals to the appropriate organs to counteract the cause of the imbalance. You may get temporary relief from the symptoms but the underlying condition will worsen because you have practically blocked the body's self-healing process.

Self - healing is an automatic process. What it means it clicks right into action without conscious thought. In fact you can't stop it from happening even if you wanted to. Even without your awareness the body automatically directs blood to your wound, cells start replicating to replace permanently damaged cells, and even determine when to stop cell replication. Interestingly, most of this occurs while you sleep.

While your conscious mind is still wandering about in your dreams, the healing process gets going - working the biochemistry and energetic transformations necessary to repair your damaged tissues. You may wonder – if self-healing is automatic why don't we always heal? Why aren't we always in perfect health?

The answer is simple. We said it before and we are saying it again – it is because we tend to erect barriers to our own healing. Worse, we refuse to read the symptoms of disease as the body's cries for help even suppressing them with medication which makes the situation worse. We don't realize that many "symptoms of disease" are manifestations of our body's attempt to heal itself.

For example, people with serious Candida overgrow will naturally experience acid reflux the main symptom of which is heartburn. Normally, a doctor will misguidedly prescribe medication for heartburn. You get temporary relief for the heartburn but in the meantime the Candida overgrowth remains undetected and uncured up to a point that it is able to wreck havoc and penetrate the intestinal walls to get into the bloodstream.

The acid reflux itself is not a disease but a cry for help - calling our attention to the fact that there exists an army of Candida yeasts that are fermenting and releasing dangerous toxins into our bloodstream. Another good example of this is high blood pressure. You may not have realized it but high blood pressure is really caused by blood that's too thick and viscous to flow freely through the body's tiny capillaries. For proper blood circulation as well as to ensure the thick and tacky blood reaches every cell, the heart has to exert more effort and pump a lot harder than normal. Remember, if the cells that don't receive blood they will die. The problem is as the heart pumps harder the blood pressure also rises.

Normal, healthy blood is not thick or viscous meaning it will flow more freely through the tiny capillaries with less friction. If the blood is properly nourished with the right fatty acids and adequately hydrated as normal, healthy blood should be then the heart does not have to pump hard to make sure blood circulates throughout the body - so the blood pressure also automatically drops.

Western medicine erroneously diagnoses "high blood pressure" as a disease by itself for which medications are meant. And this high blood pressure is attacked with drugs that artificially lower blood pressure by forcing artery walls to relax. But as the blood pressure drops, the thick, viscous blood is unable to reach all the body cells it needs to reach. The problem with the thick, viscous blood remains a problem while another problem – the problem with poor blood circulation – starts creating more serious concerns.

Symptoms such as high blood pressure and acid reflux are our body's ways of telling us to address the underlying causes of the condition. With high blood pressure, the condition may only need more water and more omega-3 fatty acids to normalize blood pressure. As the blood becomes more hydrated and free to flow throughout the circulatory system blood pressure normalizes.

Our body knows all this. Unfortunately, Western doctors know none of it or refuse to know any of it.

They treat High Blood Pressure and Acid Reflux as diseases - virtually ignoring whatever underlying causes might be creating these two measurable symptom. They fail to recognize the fact that High Blood Pressure and Acid Reflux are merely symptoms of something else that your body is attempting to balance.

Western medicine misdiagnose practically all physical symptoms of illnesses. If we wish to be healthy, we must learn to learn how to activate our body's innate healing potential. And in order for us to activate our body's innate healing potential we must learn to listen to what your body is really telling us by way of the symptoms.

We must be able to recognize the underlying conditions that produced these cries for help instead of immediately intervening with medications and/or surgeries. For example, difficulty in breathing may simply indicate dehydration. High blood pressure may be a sign of poor diet (lack of Omega 3 fats) and dehydration resulting in thick, viscous blood.

7: The Gut Is Where Everything Begins

You really don't need drugs to totally eliminate acid reflux completely. What you do need is to restore the natural balance and optimal function of your gut. There is no way you can achieve good health until your gut flora is optimized because it is through the gut flora that the body is able to absorb the much needed nutrients it requires.

Gut health is definitely critical to overall health. As Hippocrates said 2,000 years ago – "All diseases begin in the gut." True enough, we are now beginning to realize that an unhealthy gut is an aggravating factor that ultimately leads to the development of a wide range of diseases from diabetes, to obesity, to rheumatoid arthritis, to autism spectrum disorder, to depression and to chronic fatigue syndrome.

On the other hand, a healthy gut means good health. And as far as gut health is concerned we are actually looking at the status of two things – the "gut flora" or intestinal micro-biota and the gut barrier.

Our gut is host to about 100 trillion microorganisms. That is such a mind bungling number too large for the human brain to comprehend. But much more mind bungling is the fact that the human gut has ten times more bacteria than all the human cells in the entire human body. It is home to over 500 known bacterial species and comprises over 75% of our immune system. Like a healthy garden that needs healthy soil, the gut flora has to remain fertile to retain its diversity and health to promote normal gastric functions.

While a healthy gut flora provides protection from infection, promotes normal gastrointestinal function, and regulates metabolism, a deregulated (unhealthy) gut flora is almost always linked to a wide array of debilitating diseases.

Certain modern lifestyle features like the use of antibiotics, birth control pills, and NSAIDs; consumption of processed foods and diets that are high in refined sugar and carbohydrates; low fiber diets; Chronic stress; dietary toxins such as wheat and seed oils; and chronic infections – actually harm the human gut resulting in unhealthy gut flora.

Particularly destructive to the gut flora is the use of antibiotics. Recent studies have shown that the use of antibiotics results in the rapid and profound loss of diversity and a drastic change composition of the gut flora landscape.

The gut barrier on the other hand serves as the gatekeeper that decides what gets in and what stays out of the human body. The gut is a hollow tube that passes from the mouth to the anus. Anything that goes in the mouth that is not digested passes right out to the other end. The main function of the gut is to prevent toxins and foreign substances from entering the body and the gut barrier plays a vital role in making this happen.

However, if and when the gut barrier becomes permeable (due to infection or inflammation) large protein molecules will then be able to penetrate and pass on all the way through into the bloodstream. But as soon as they get there, they will be promptly dealt with as an invader and attacked with an auto immune response just like any foreign body.

These auto immune responses are what ultimately develop into autoimmune diseases like diabetes – meaning this is where and how autoimmune diseases get their start – large protein molecules able to penetrate the gut barrier and into the blood stream and promptly attacked by the auto immune system!

Clearly, the health of your gut determines what nutrients are absorbed and how much toxins, allergens and microbes are kept out – which in effect links it directly to the health of the individual. Gut health is defined as the optimal digestion, absorption and assimilation of food – tall order meant to keep you healthy – dependent on how it is able to maintain and retain balance in a diverse and interdependent ecosystem.

If maintaining the balance between the good and the bad among the five hundred species and 100 trillion microorganisms that includes bacteria and viruses in your gut is not a tall order I don't know what is. The gut operates like a huge chemical factory constantly preoccupied with helping you churn and digest your food, producing vitamins, helping regulate hormones, filtering toxins and producing healing compounds to keep your gut healthy.

If it falters and allows too many of the bad microorganisms like bad bacteria, parasites, or yeasts to overgrow, or if *not enough* of the good bacteria like lactobacillus or bifidobacteria is in the gut – then expect serious damage to befall on your health. Once again, as Hippocrates clearly described it 2,000 years ago – "*All diseases begin in the gut.*"

Cleansing – The most Important Secret of All

Most illnesses occur when the body is unable to remove all the excessive amounts of toxins that get lodged into your cell walls, tissues, hormone receptors, bones, and even cell surfaces over time. More often than not a disease sets in the minute toxins are able to penetrate your system so much so that it's often too late when symptoms appear because by then damage has been done.

That is why we need to cleanse – to clean our system of all the garbage that has accumulated in our body since the day we were born. Believe it or not, people are still carrying with them the remnants of bad food and thoughts from childhood. Cleansing our body of all the toxins and garbage residue is the secret to staying healthy. The body needs to get rid of not just undigested food wastes but also millions of dead cells every day. That's right, dead cells are also toxic and they need to be removed from our system fast. About 100 pounds of these toxic dead cells are sent to our bowels every year and if we don't cleanse properly all the way down to the colon on a regular basis, we may end up accumulating more toxic waste than our system can handle.

Disease sets in only when the body is in a state of disharmony (imbalance) due to either excessive toxicity or nutrient deficiency. The symptoms produced by the disease indicates that something had gone wrong and that there is an imbalance that puts you at risk and needs to be corrected.

Cleansing is like rebuilding an old house where you have to strip it down to its barest structure - scraping away every termite and every bit of rusted nail. Similarly, we have to strip our bodies down to deepest abyss of our colons to clean out all the toxic garbage that have been accumulating in our body since the day we were born.

The internal cleansing process of removing toxins is more popularly known as detoxification. It aims not only to rid the body of accumulated toxic waste but also to restore the body's state of balance with the right nutrition. Cleansing will result in more than 90% of illnesses being healed by the body itself.

In other words, cleansing is the best way to eradicate any and all illness and disease you may have. By eliminating the toxins that have built up in your system, you should be able to cure as well as prevent illness and disease from occurring in the future. On top of that, detoxification can immediately increase energy, help you lose weight, and eliminate depression and anxiety. As an added bonus, cleansing may even reverse the aging process.

There are 7 basic cleanses that you should do. They are:

1. A colon cleanse,
2. A liver/gallbladder cleanse
3. A kidney/bladder cleanse
4. A heavy metal cleanse
5. A parasite cleanse
6. A Candida cleanse
7. A full-body fat tissue/lymphatic cleanse

Needless to say, we live in a highly toxic world which means it is almost impossible to totally eliminate toxins from our body. However, we have the power to dramatically reduce the amount of toxins entering our body.

We just have to make sure we are getting proper amounts of nutrition – e.g. the right amounts of vitamins, minerals, enzymes, cofactors, and life-sustaining "energy". Our system has to be able to assimilate these vital nutrients so that they can be utilized in maintaining our health.

8: Plugging the Gaping Hole

Once you stop doing the things that are causing your symptoms and disease, then you have in fact practically "cured" your disease. One of the things they don't want you to know is how to plug the gaping hole that allows toxins to get into our system. We must help the liver get rid of whatever toxins are already inside our systems, otherwise the liver will be tied up with getting rid of new toxins while the old toxins continue to build up to a point that the stored toxins start causing damage even to the fat cells thus affecting their metabolic capabilities.

Where do the toxins come from and how do we plug the gaping hole?

Toxins and other poisonous substances foreign to our bodily system find their way into our bodies through the food we eat, through the water we drink, and even through the air we breathe. They come in various forms from toxic residues of antibiotics injected into livestock and poultry to fend off diseases, from the growth hormones they are fed to insure their growth, from the industrial feeds produced from genetically modified corn meal and grains.

They get embedded in the meat of the farm animals we buy from the supermarket. They come in the form of fertilizer, herbicide, and pesticide residues that remain in the farm produce such as fruits and vegetables. They can come in the form of high concentrations of sodium and sugar in the water we drink and the processed foods we purchase. Toxins may also come in the form of environmental pollutants in the air we inhale.

Environmental toxins have been dubbed as silent killers because they get into our bodies undetected and wreck havoc on our immune system. These invisible killers come in the food we eat, water we drink, and the air we breathe such as antibiotics, growth hormones, and industrial feed residues that become embedded in the meat we buy from the supermarket; fertilizer, herbicide, and pesticide residues in the farm produce; high concentrations of sodium in the water we drink and the processed foods we purchase; toxic industrial by products in the air we inhale and the toxic materials we handle. Somehow, they get into our systems on a regular basis keeping our immune systems perpetually pre-occupied with the task of cleansing our blood of these toxins.

The only way to plug the gaping hole and prevent further toxin build up in our bodies is to eat only natural, whole foods – unprocessed, organically grown, grass fed, pasture-raised or caught from the wild.

Our First Line of Treatment – Natural, Unprocessed Foods and Probiotics

Ultimately, the answer to heartburn and acid indigestion is to restore your natural gastric balance and function. Certainly, eating large amounts of processed foods heavy in sugars and carbohydrates is guaranteed to exacerbate acid reflux. The presence of sugar tilts the bacterial balance in your gut in favor of the bad bacteria and harmful yeast.

What you want to do get on a diet plan that basically eliminates the food sources of environmental toxins - effectively plugging one of the entry points of these silent killers. You'll want to eat a lot of vegetables and other high-quality, ideally organic, unprocessed foods. Also, you may want to eliminate foods which triggers acid reflux symptoms from your diet – such as caffeine, alcohol, and nicotine products.

Avoid 'Frankenfoods'

Giant agribusiness have genetically engineered food and food sources as well as food ingredients and bombarded the market with them.

These giant agribusiness interests have practically taken a strangle hold on us by making us totally dependent on the so-called 'Frankenfoods' or genetically engineered food products which they have produced. Hoodwinking us into believing they are totally safe and feeding health authorities with questionable safety studies, they have practically flooded the consumer market with food products using genetically modified food sources they have created in their labs.

Genetically-modified foods (*labeled in jest as 'Frankenfoods' by its critics*) have taken over much of our food supply without us being aware of it. They are used as ingredients in producing processed foods or as feeds for grain-fed cattle the end products of which find their way into our dining tables through the meat we eat along with the artificial genes they have created.

The sad part is despite the claims of the manufacturers and the shady endorsements by health authorities that they are relatively safe for human consumption an increasing number of independent research studies persistently link the continued consumption of these genetically modified foods to the high incidence of allergies, sterility, infant mortality, childhood illness, organ defects, and even cancer.

If you don't have any idea of what 'Frankenfoods' are, below is a short list of the most popular ones that has become very much a part of our daily existence.

Genetically Modified Alfalfa

If you think you are not consuming Alfalfa, think again. The natural Alfalfa is an important forage crop cultivated for use as livestock fodder. Since the Romans and the Greek era, Alfalfa has been used by farmers to feed their cows. They have however been genetically modified by giant agri-business interests like Monsanto so that they can produce higher yield and at the same time be resistant to herbicides such as Round up (*a popular herbicide used by farmers to kill the weeds*).

The genetically modified Alfalfa along with its transgenes (*artificial genes*) gets into our system through the meat and dairy products we eat and God knows what kind of havoc it can do to our system. Even in its natural form, Alfalfa is known to contain *phytoestrogens* which are basically estrogen blockers that cause reduced fertility in mammals. The Alfalfa seeds meanwhile contain the amino acid canavine which interacts with another amino acid arginine resulting in the synthesizing of dysfunctional proteins which are toxic to humans and produce lupus-like symptoms.

Aspartame

Aspartame is more popularly known as *Nutrasweet*. This is a popular artificial sweetener used in most food processing applications including beverages. Aspartame has been established as a neurotoxin which disrupts brain functions and our immune systems. Despite endorsements by nutritionists and health authorities to its safety, there is mounting evidence that shows that aspartame aggravates insulin sensitivity and causes a lot of other health disorders. In fact one comprehensive study even linked leukemia and non-Hodgkin's Lymphoma to continued aspartame consumption.

Ranch-raised Beef

The main reason why Paleo recommends organic meat from pasture-raised, grass fed livestock is because ranch-raised live stocks are fed not only with genetically modified alfalfa but also with genetically modified corn and soy meal. They are also injected with all sorts of things that to ensure their health and faster growth such as growth hormones, antibiotics, and vaccines which sadly also find their way into our bodies through the food we eat.

Canola Oil

Almost 90% of the canola produced in the world has been genetically-modified in order to weather the effects of herbicides (*particularly glyphosate more popularly known as Round Up*) during planting. Aside from the transgenes, large quantities of the herbicide can be found in the finished canola oil products.

Corn, corn meal, and Corn Starch

With almost all the corn planted in the U.S. being genetically-modified to resist herbicides and pesticides, you can be sure that all the products and ingredients made from modified corn carry trans genes too as well as traces of the pesticides and herbicides used. The gory part is genetically modified corn products are used in almost all processed and packaged foods. These include Corn oil, corn flour, corn starch, corn syrup, corn meal, gluten, and sweeteners such as fructose, dextrose, and glucose. They are used in making baked goods, fried foods, snack foods, confectionery, special purpose foods, edible oil products, and soft drinks.

Vitamins

Take a second look at the vitamins you are taking. They may have been manufactured from genetically modified plant sources or may have used genetically modified ingredients as carriers. For example, Vitamin C is usually made from *Frankencorn* while vitamin E is made from *Frankensoy*.

Enzymes

Almost all the enzymes used for food processing come from genetically modified products like the enzymes used to prevent egg products from spoiling; enzymes that removes the bitter taste from beer; enzymes that improve the clarity of fruit juices; enzymes to help milk clotting for making cheese; enzymes to speed the rise of bread dough; and enzymes used to manufacture many food supplements.

Ice Cream

One thing you should be wary of when you buy ice cream is whether or not it contains several genetically-modified ingredients like corn starch, high fructose corn syrup, and milk from cows that were injected with bovine growth hormone (rBGH). The bovine growth hormone is injected into cows to make them grow faster and produce more milk. In studies made on rBGH by the University of Vermont as commissioned by agribusiness giant Monsanto, five calves were born from cows injected with rBGH with rare deformities that were never seen before. This was however downplayed. Can you imagine if rBGH filters into your system from the ice cream you eat?

Infant Formula

Manufacturers of infant formula who used frankenfood ingredients like genetically modified soy and milk from rBGH injected cows may be unmindful of the health hazards they bring. You should be wary of this before you buy your next infant formula.

Margarine and Shortening

Contrary to the general belief margarine and shortening made from vegetable blends and canola are not healthy. Most of the ingredients used are genetically modified.

Milk

Milk from cows injected with bovine growth hormone (rBGH) may contain blood and pus as a result of infection resulting from the rBGH injection. Studies have shown that cows injected with rBGH become highly susceptible to infections and those which becomes infected may have blood and pus in their milk along with the rBGH and any antibiotics that may have been injected into the cows to prevent the spread of the infection.

Soy and Lecithin

Almost all of the soybean crops planted are genetically-modified soy which means all soy products including Lecithin may have harmful trans genes. Lecithin is normally used as a thickener by food processors and packaged food manufacturers.

Sugar Beets

Most sugar beets from which 35% of the global supply of refined white sugar comes from are also mostly genetically modified. So, you not only risk having a spike in your blood sugar levels but also the risk having artificial genes filtered into your system along with fertilizer, herbicide, and pesticide residues.

Tomatoes

Tomatoes have been genetically modified so they will have longer shelf life. They have a reversed DNA sequence so that they won't soften even if stored longer. They however have much less nutrients than organic tomatoes on top of the modified genes they pass on to us.

Vegetable Oil

Most, if not all the "vegetable oil" sold in supermarkets are refined from genetically-modified soybean oils, canola, corn, or cotton seed.

What you should eat

Fruits and Vegetables

Ordinary fruits and vegetables are not only laden with fertilizers, herbicides, and pesticides many of them have been genetically modified too. Sadly, they have been linked to cancer and to disorders in the endocrine and nervous system because of the toxins they carry. The toxins find their way into our systems when we eat these fruits and vegetables.

We recommend eating only high quality organic fruits and vegetables. Look for the 'USDA Certified Organic' on the label. This is how you can be sure the fruits and vegetables you buy are free of insecticides, chemical fertilizers, pesticides, and herbicides. You can also be sure they have not been genetically engineered or have undergone irradiation.

Animal Protein Sources

We recommend organic, grass-fed meat from pasture raised livestock or wild game meat for your animal protein sources. Ordinary meat contains toxins stored in their fat such as residues of the antibiotics, growth hormones, grain based industrial feeds, and vitamins that are given to the livestock to ensure their growth to gain more profits.

If certified organic, grass-fed meat is unavailable in your area, buy lean meat instead. The animal toxins are likely to be in the animal fat since like humans, animals too store the toxins in their fat cells.

Healthy Fats

Fat is essential in forming new cells and strengthening cell membranes. However, there are beneficial fats and poor quality fats. Logically, the poor quality creates poor quality cells which subsequently lead to serious health problems. The worst type of poor quality fats are the trans fats from highly processed oils like canola and vegetable oil. Trans fats are created artificially through the hydrogenation of vegetable oil to make the oil last longer without spoiling. Food processors prefer to use hydrogenated vegetable oil not only to extend the shelf life of their processed food products but also because of the texture and quality of their finished products.

Trans fat (*also known as trans fatty acids*) have been shown to raise the level of the Low Density Lipoproteins (*bad cholesterol*) and lower the level of the High Density Lipoproteins (*good cholesterol*) in the blood thus increasing the risk of heart disease.

If you are concerned with your health and long term well-being, then this is the ideal diet for you. This is much more than just an eating plan. It is a completely unique lifestyle that requires drastic changes in the way you currently live your life – particularly in your outlook on the kinds of food you eat. It means giving up your favorite comfort foods in exchange for eating food that are practically unprocessed and comes in their most natural form possible. It means eating healthy and keeping the toxins out.

Probiotics

The last but not the least important thing you must do is to make sure you're getting enough beneficial bacteria from your diet. You need to help maintain the bacterial balance your bowel flora and eliminate *H. pylori* bacteria naturally without using antibiotics. The best way to do this is to get your probiotics from fermented foods such as yogurt and sauerkraut. If you are not much into fermented foods, you can try taking probiotic supplements on a regular basis.

Conclusion

The material in this book is provided for educational and informational purposes only. It should not be used as a substitute for a visit to a health care provider for an appropriate professional consultation.

There is always that possibility that the symptoms you have may be caused by something other than simple acid reflux – which means adopting the remedies contained in this book without consulting a health professional could possibly delay finding the right prognosis for your condition. So, please refer the recommendations and opinions contained in this book pertaining to your specific symptoms and health condition to your physician or health care provider before applying or adopting any of them.

The author, producers, publishers and narrator, shall neither be liable nor be in any way responsible to any person or entity with respect to any loss, damage, sickness or injury caused or alleged to be caused directly or indirectly by the information contained in this book.